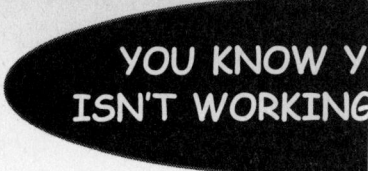

YOU KNOW YOUR DIET ISN'T WORKING WHEN...

Emma Burgess

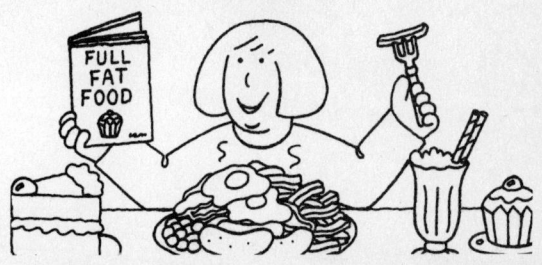

SUMMERSDALE

Copyright © Summersdale Publishers Ltd 2001

All rights reserved

No part of this book may be reproduced by any means, nor transmitted, nor translated into a machine language without the written permission of the publisher

Summersdale Publishers Ltd
46 West Street
Chichester
PO19 1RP

www.summersdale.com

ISBN 1 84024 196 9

Printed and bound in Great Britain

Text by Emma Burgess
Cartoons by Kate Taylor

You know your diet isn't working when . . .

YOU KNOW YOUR DIET ISN'T WORKING WHEN . . .

Your arse needs its own passport.

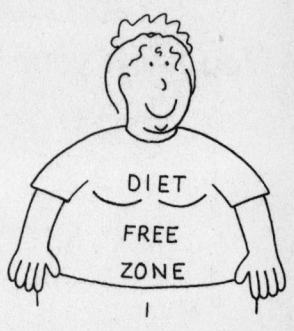

YOU KNOW YOUR DIET ISN'T WORKING WHEN . . .

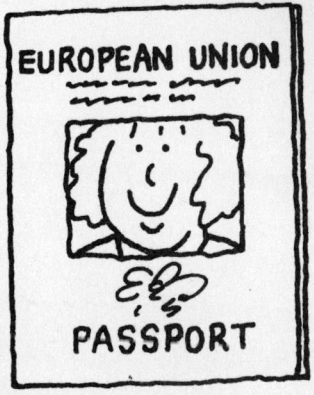 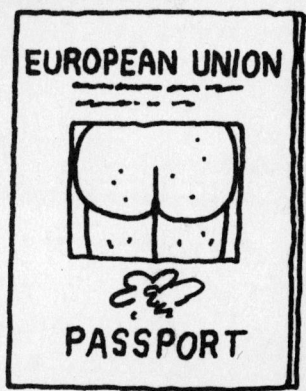

YOU KNOW YOUR DIET ISN'T WORKING WHEN . . .

You own a couple of boob tubes, but you wear them as legwarmers.

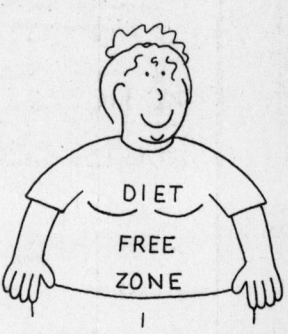

YOU KNOW YOUR DIET ISN'T WORKING WHEN . . .

You entertain at kids' parties...as the bouncy castle.

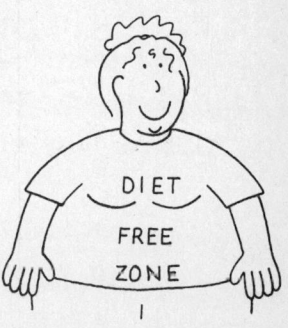

YOU KNOW YOUR DIET ISN'T WORKING WHEN . . .

Lycra is for you the best invention since sliced bread.

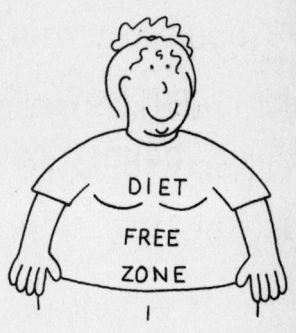

YOU KNOW YOUR DIET ISN'T WORKING WHEN . . .

On second thoughts, sliced bread (preferably with butter and chocolate spread) is far better than Lycra.

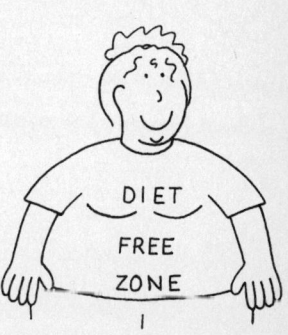

YOU KNOW YOUR DIET ISN'T WORKING WHEN . . .

Friends notice your generosity...with your portions at least.

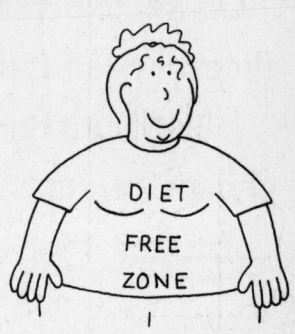

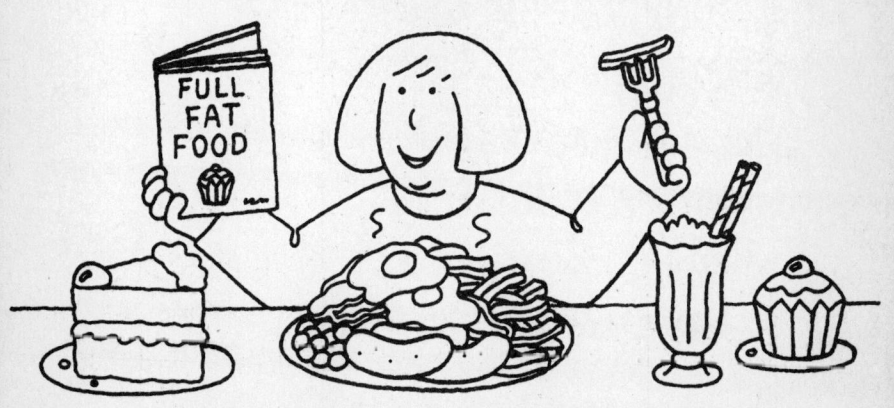

YOU KNOW YOUR DIET ISN'T WORKING WHEN . . .

You can't see your toes. The only time you're aware of their existence is when they send you a postcard.

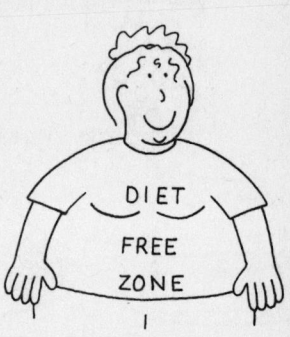

YOU KNOW YOUR DIET ISN'T WORKING WHEN . . .

You join the Navy...
as an anchor.

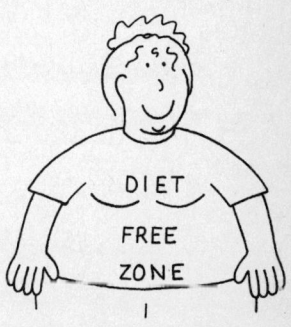

YOU KNOW YOUR DIET ISN'T WORKING WHEN . . .

You no longer wear large pants ironically.

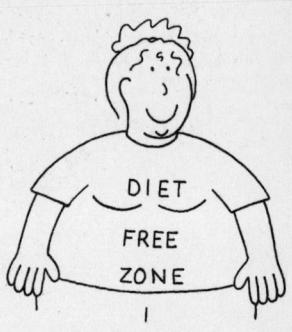

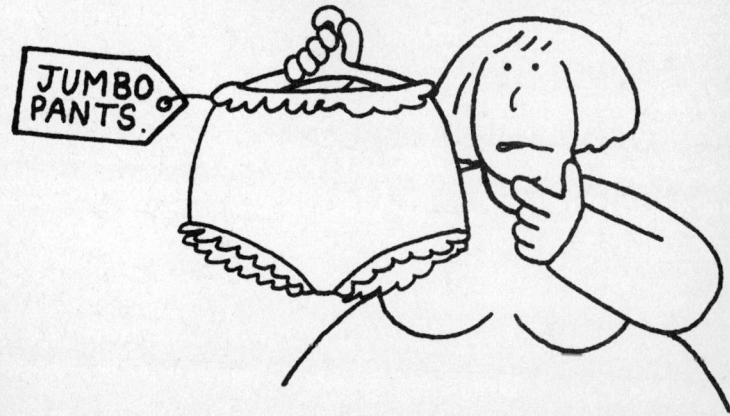

YOU KNOW YOUR DIET ISN'T WORKING WHEN . . .

Nosy but well-meaning strangers often ask you whether it's a girl or a boy. Or a football team.

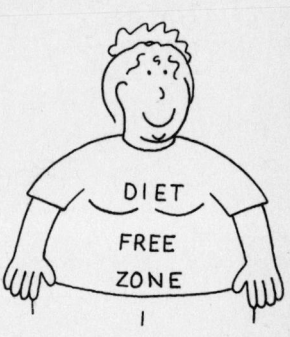

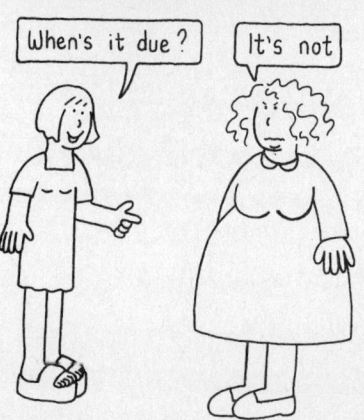

YOU KNOW YOUR DIET ISN'T WORKING WHEN . . .

You have an operation to extend your arm length so that you can wipe the whole of your bum.

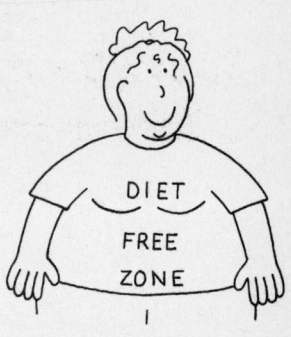

YOU KNOW YOUR DIET ISN'T WORKING WHEN . . .

To you, Dawn French looks anorexic.

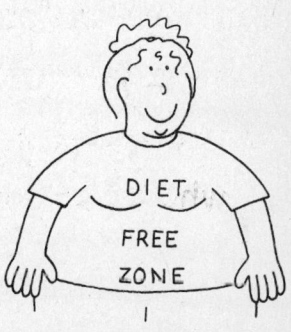

YOU KNOW YOUR DIET ISN'T WORKING WHEN . . .

You spend a lot of your time in tracksuits. Ironic, huh?

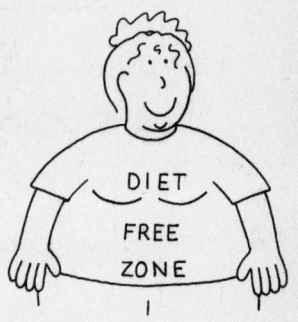

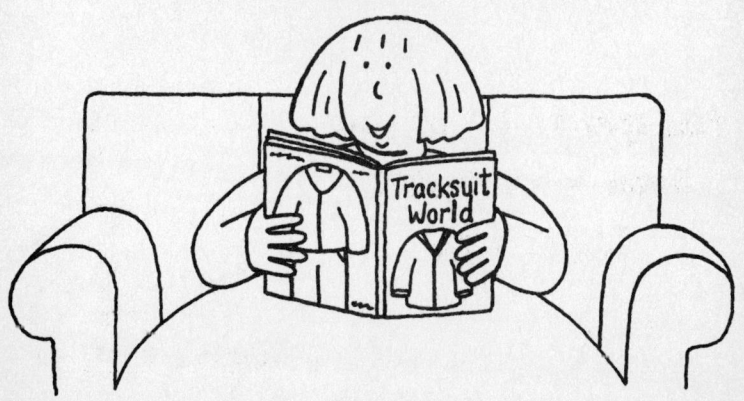

YOU KNOW YOUR DIET ISN'T WORKING WHEN . . .

You have more folds than a prize-winning example of origami.

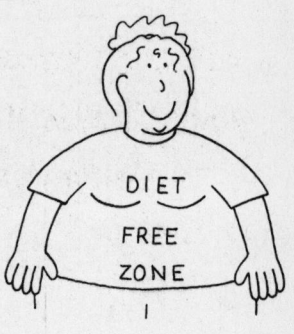

YOU KNOW YOUR DIET ISN'T WORKING WHEN . . .

You can't even fit into your Slendertone belt anymore.

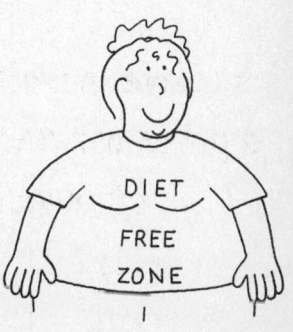

YOU KNOW YOUR DIET ISN'T WORKING WHEN . . .

You wish kaftans would come back into fashion.

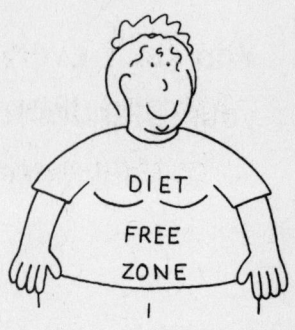

YOU KNOW YOUR DIET ISN'T WORKING WHEN . . .

You have a higher fat content than an EU butter mountain.

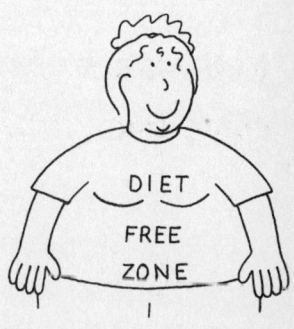

YOU KNOW YOUR DIET ISN'T WORKING WHEN . . .

You part exchange your 2-seater sofa for a 3-seater even though you live alone.

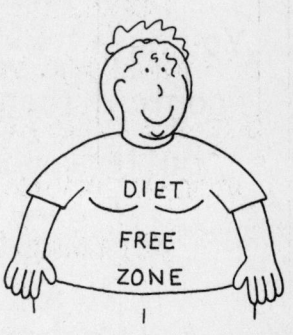

YOU KNOW YOUR DIET ISN'T WORKING WHEN . . .

People never acknowledge your size but are always keen to comment on your 'lovely personality'.

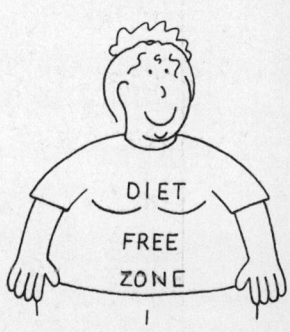

YOU KNOW YOUR DIET ISN'T WORKING WHEN . . .

You attend 'bounce classes' not 'step'.

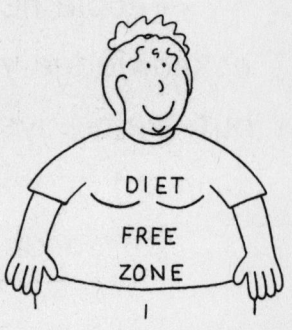

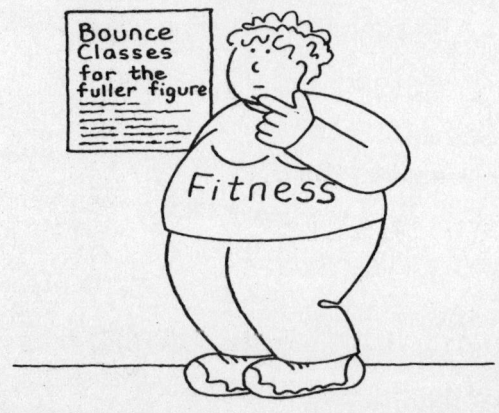

YOU KNOW YOUR DIET ISN'T WORKING WHEN . . .

You're invited to take part in a weight loss TV programme. Actually, you're the only person in it...there isn't room for anyone else.

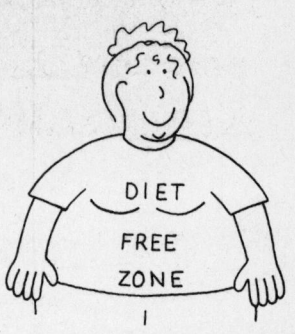

YOU KNOW YOUR DIET ISN'T WORKING WHEN . . .

In the school panto, you were cast as the front and back end of a horse.

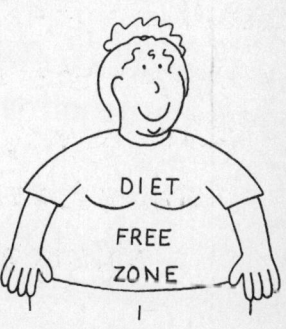

YOU KNOW YOUR DIET ISN'T WORKING WHEN . . .

Your friends are constantly asking you 'who ate all the pies?' (Just to set the record straight, it was you.)

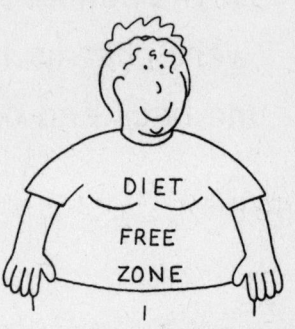

YOU KNOW YOUR DIET ISN'T WORKING WHEN . . .

Your Sunday roast is the whole herd.

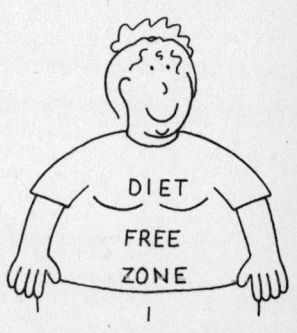

YOU KNOW YOUR DIET ISN'T WORKING WHEN . . .

Your passport photo has to be taken with a wide angled lense.

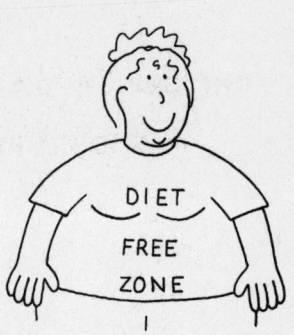

YOU KNOW YOUR DIET ISN'T WORKING WHEN . . .

As a child, you wore a trough at meal times and not a bib.

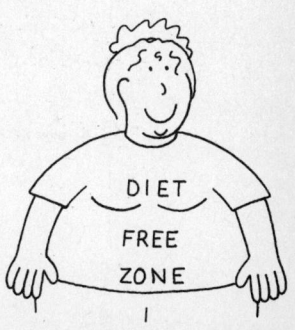

YOU KNOW YOUR DIET ISN'T WORKING WHEN . . .

Your ear lobes have cellulite. So does your cellulite.

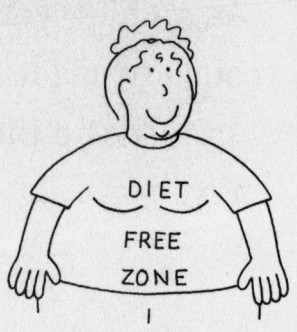

YOU KNOW YOUR DIET ISN'T WORKING WHEN . . .

At school, your class did a geography field trip on you...and 3 pupils never returned from their picnic at your Hanging Rock.

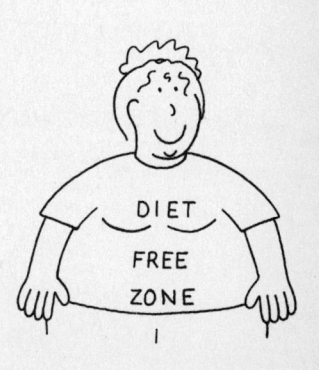

YOU KNOW YOUR DIET ISN'T WORKING WHEN . . .

You have bras specially made...to support all eight breasts.

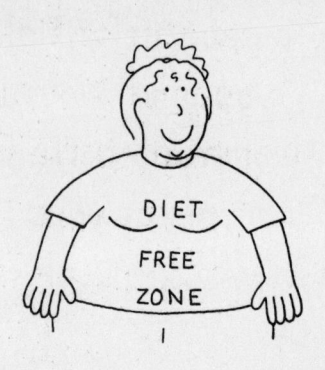

YOU KNOW YOUR DIET ISN'T WORKING WHEN . . .

You tell people that you're having to put weight on for a film role.

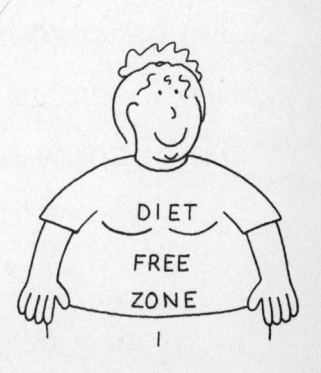

YOU KNOW YOUR DIET ISN'T WORKING WHEN . . .

Your partner padlocks your fridge...but you soon learn to enjoy the taste of just plain old cutlery.

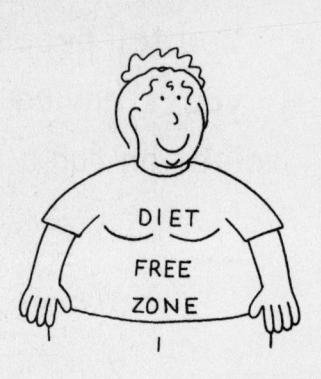

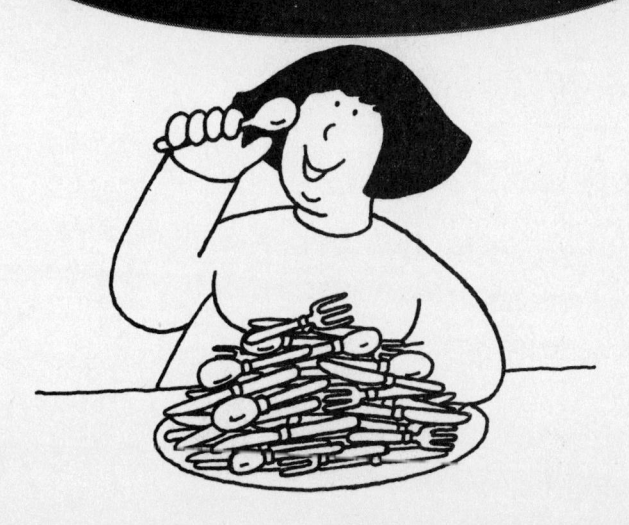

YOU KNOW YOUR DIET ISN'T WORKING WHEN . . .

Your dress size reads more like a serial number.

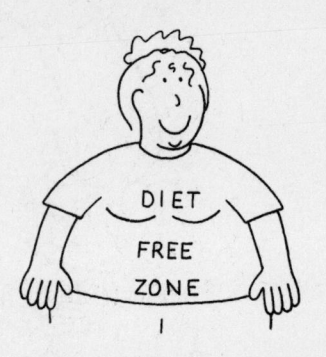

YOU KNOW YOUR DIET ISN'T WORKING WHEN . . .

You have more contours than the Pennines.

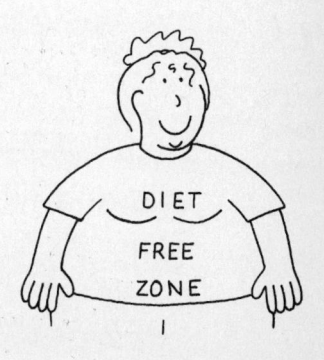

YOU KNOW YOUR DIET ISN'T WORKING WHEN . . .

You've had your teeth removed as part of a weight loss programme. Thank goodness for straws and full-fat milkshakes.

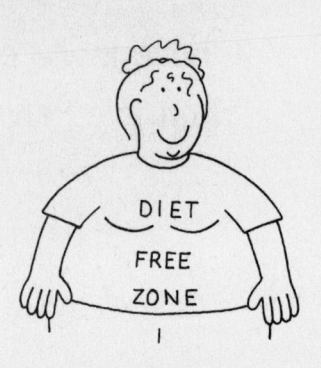

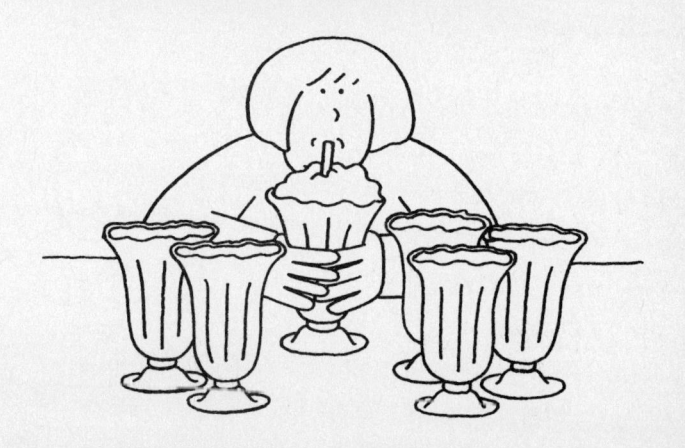

YOU KNOW YOUR DIET ISN'T WORKING WHEN . . .

You're idea of a diet is having single cream on your deep-fried Mars bar, not double.

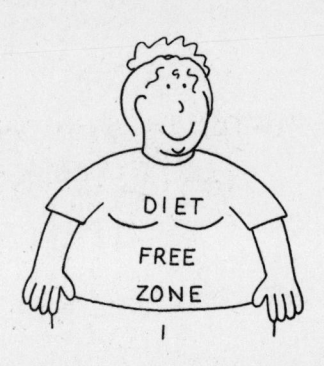

YOU KNOW YOUR DIET ISN'T WORKING WHEN . . .

You used to have a tattoo but you can't seem to find it anymore.

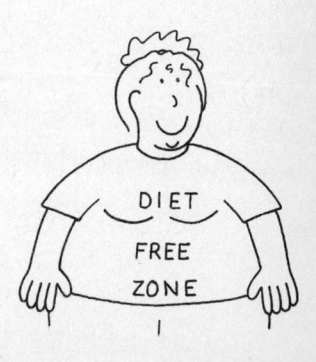

YOU KNOW YOUR DIET ISN'T WORKING WHEN . . .

You stopped weighing yourself when your special zoo-keeper's scales packed in.

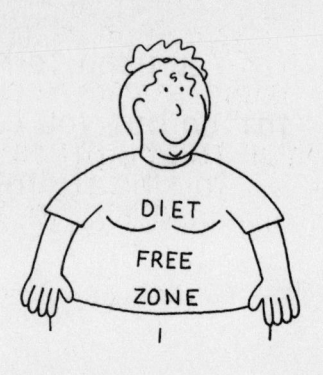

YOU KNOW YOUR DIET ISN'T WORKING WHEN . . .

The owner of your local supermarket campaigns for the reintroduction of ration books.

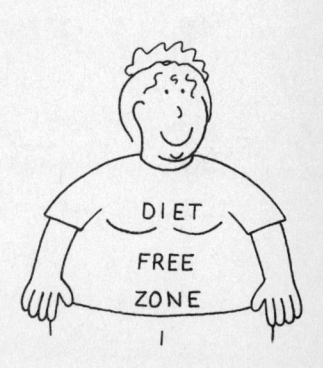

YOU KNOW YOUR DIET ISN'T WORKING WHEN . . .

Your partner leaves you, citing Black Forest Gâteaux in the divorce.

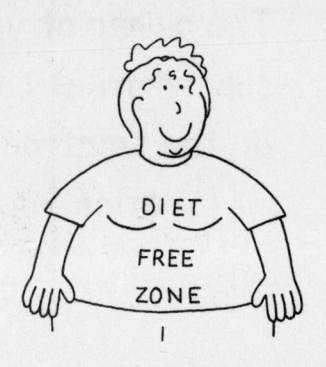

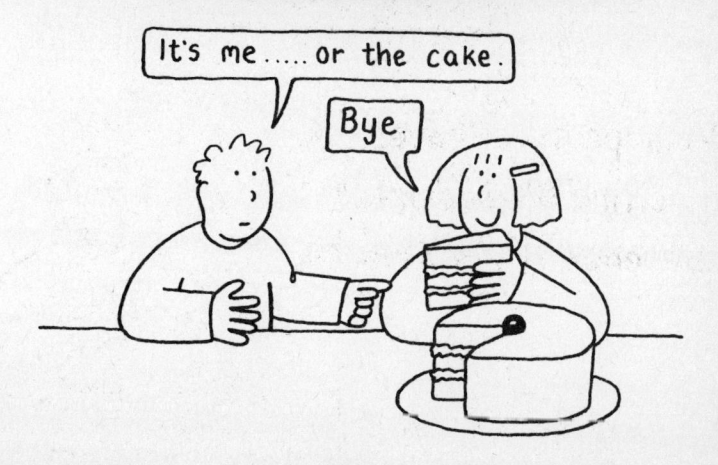

YOU KNOW YOUR DIET ISN'T WORKING WHEN . . .

You wear a clock on your wrist.

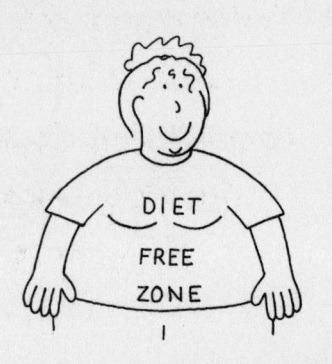

YOU KNOW YOUR DIET ISN'T WORKING WHEN . . .

You win a year's supply of confectionery in a competition. It takes you just a week to get through it all.

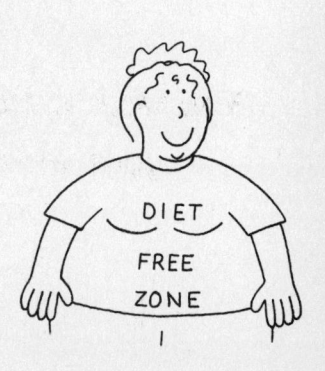

YOU KNOW YOUR DIET ISN'T WORKING WHEN . . .

You've donated money to your local Sainsbury's...so they could custom build a triple-sized trolley for your daily shop.

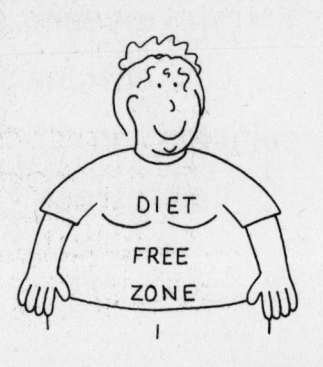

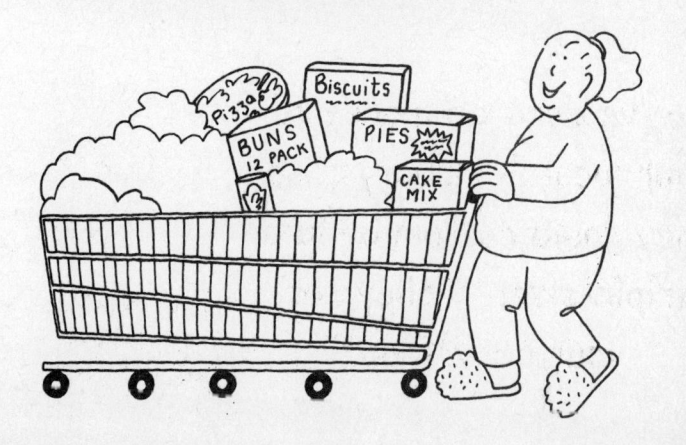

YOU KNOW YOUR DIET ISN'T WORKING WHEN . . .

You take coffee with your morning sugar.

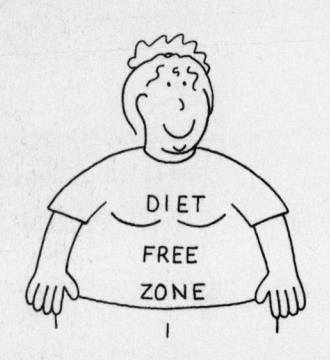

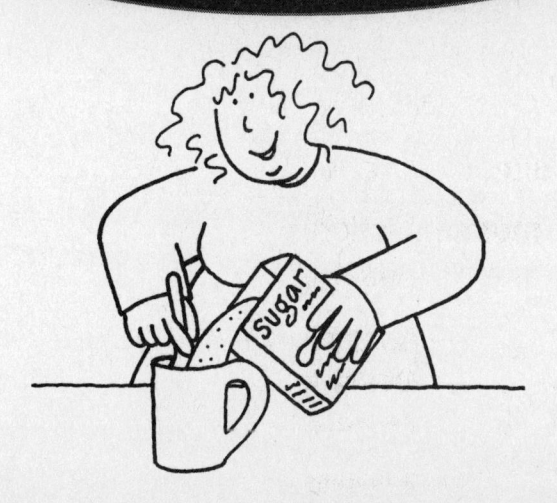

YOU KNOW YOUR DIET ISN'T WORKING WHEN . . .

The only sport you are eligible for is sumo wrestling.

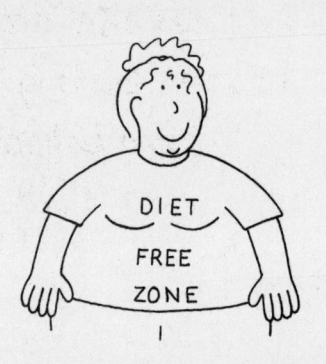

YOU KNOW YOUR DIET ISN'T WORKING WHEN . . .

Your sex life is explosive.
It's like putting a needle
in a balloon.

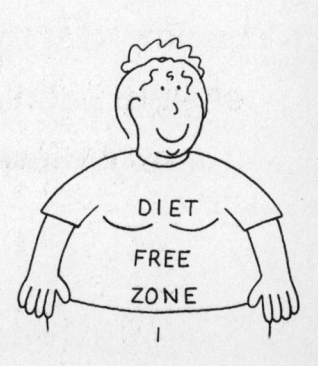

YOU KNOW YOUR DIET ISN'T WORKING WHEN . . .

At your wedding, you wear the marquee.

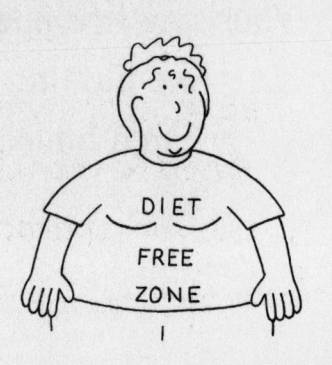

DIET FREE ZONE

YOU KNOW YOUR DIET ISN'T WORKING WHEN . . .

Your bosoms are so big that your cup size has to be interpreted in the Chinese alphabet of 3,000 characters.

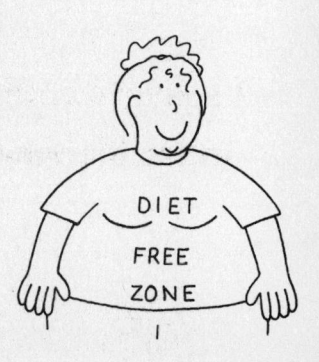

YOU KNOW YOUR DIET ISN'T WORKING WHEN . . .

You salivate when opening a tin of cat food.

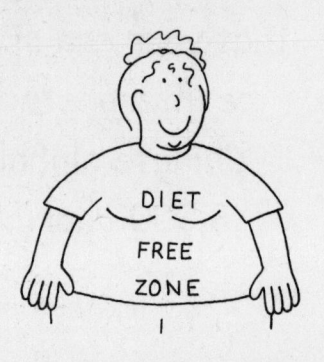

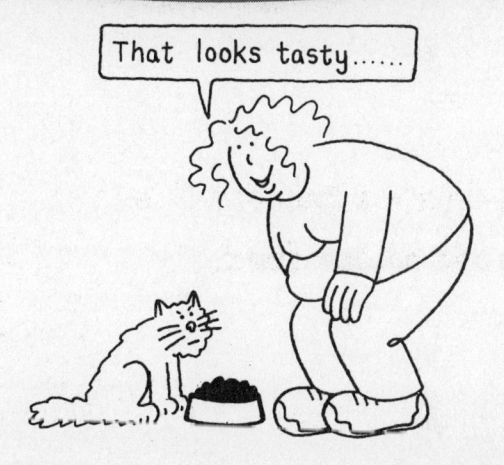

YOU KNOW YOUR DIET ISN'T WORKING WHEN . . .

You are the back-end of a bus.

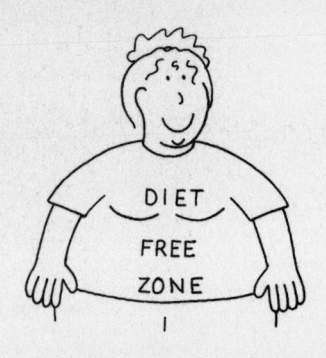

YOU KNOW YOUR DIET ISN'T WORKING WHEN . . .

You were asked to join a travelling circus...to soften the landing in case the trapeze artist falls.

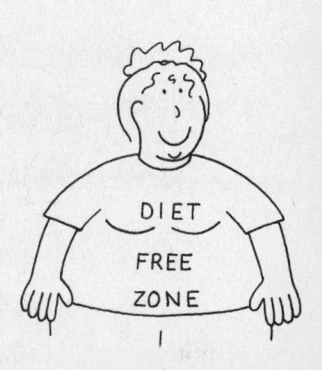

YOU KNOW YOUR DIET ISN'T WORKING WHEN . . .

Your beauty therapist can't find your bikini line anymore.

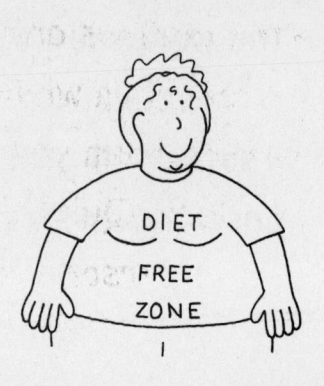

YOU KNOW YOUR DIET ISN'T WORKING WHEN . . .

You have lipo-suction and the doctors are able to fashion a whole new person from your excess lard. Quite a fat person too.

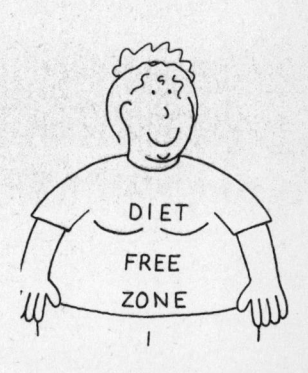

YOU KNOW YOUR DIET ISN'T WORKING WHEN . . .

Turning over in bed is trickier than a three-point turn.

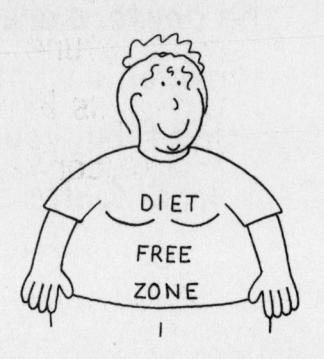

YOU KNOW YOUR DIET ISN'T WORKING WHEN . . .

You feature in the Guinness Book of Records.

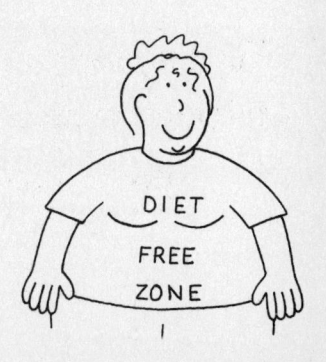

YOU KNOW YOUR DIET ISN'T WORKING WHEN . . .

You burn more calories in bending over to paint your toes than you do when walking to the corner shop (to buy a chocolate bar).

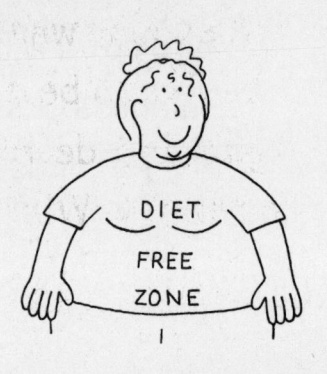

YOU KNOW YOUR DIET ISN'T WORKING WHEN . . .

You wonder what it would be like to be a size 16 again, but decide it's pie in the sky. Who said pie?

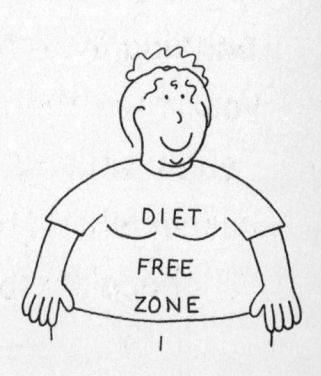

YOU KNOW YOUR DIET ISN'T WORKING WHEN . . .

You fervently believe that the secret of losing weight will one day appear on the inside of a crisp packet. Your enthusiasm in this search is frightening.

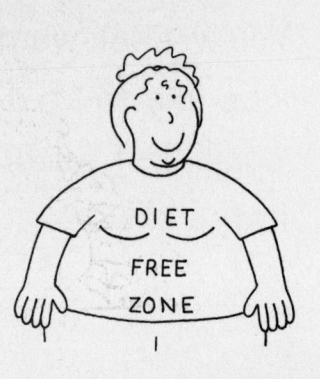

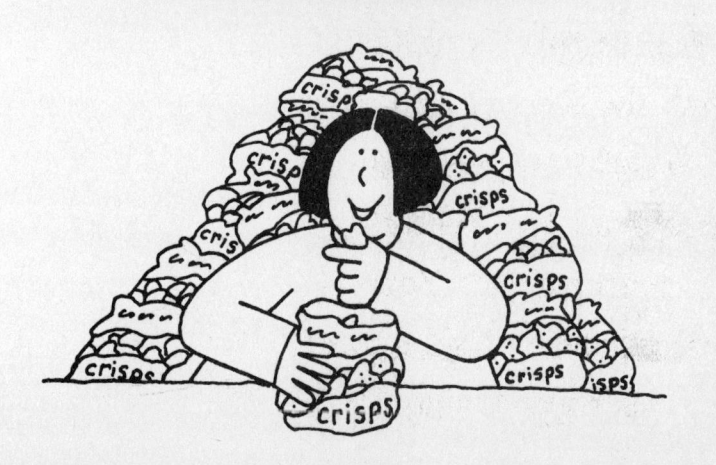

YOU KNOW YOUR DIET ISN'T WORKING WHEN . . .

You take diet suppressant tablets, but eat so many you end up getting fatter.

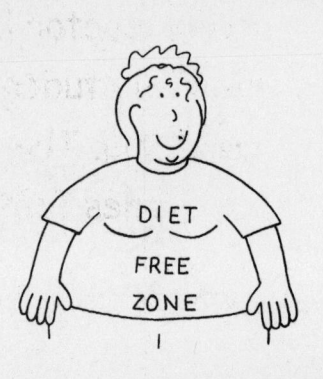

YOU KNOW YOUR DIET ISN'T WORKING WHEN . . .

Your doctor invites medical students in to meet you. The weaker ones faint.

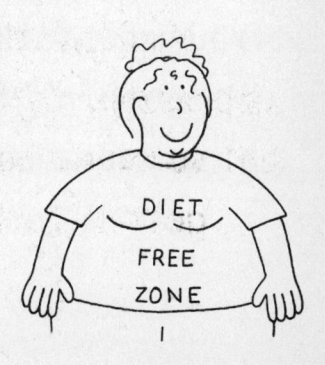

YOU KNOW YOUR DIET ISN'T WORKING WHEN . . .

You are a fat person trapped in a fatter person's body.

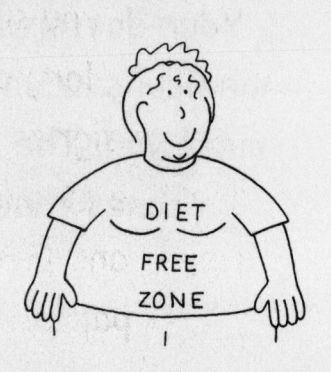

YOU KNOW YOUR DIET ISN'T WORKING WHEN...

Your husband stopped buying you saucy underwear long ago. You are resigned to a lifetime of support tights and panelled pants.

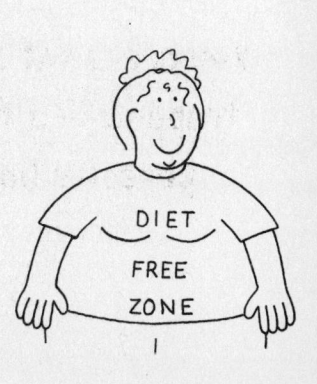

YOU KNOW YOUR DIET ISN'T WORKING WHEN . . .

You are the most popular bridesmaid – you never look better than the bride.

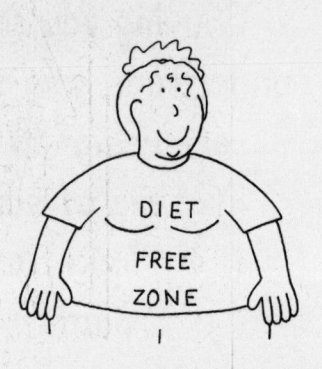

YOU KNOW YOUR DIET ISN'T WORKING WHEN . . .

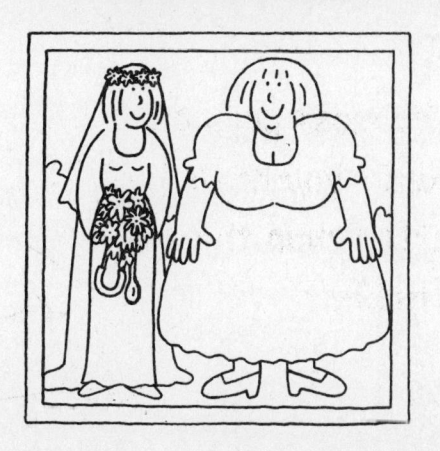

YOU KNOW YOUR DIET ISN'T WORKING WHEN . . .

You need a JCB to get you into your bikini.

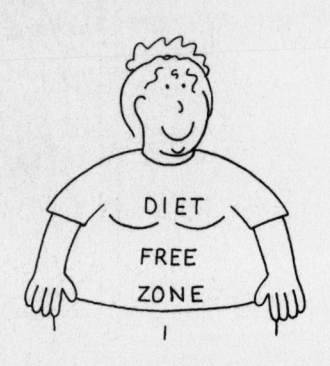

YOU KNOW YOUR DIET ISN'T WORKING WHEN . . .

You are asked to appear in a WeightWatchers ad campaign, but they have to sack you because you break all the rules...and the scales.

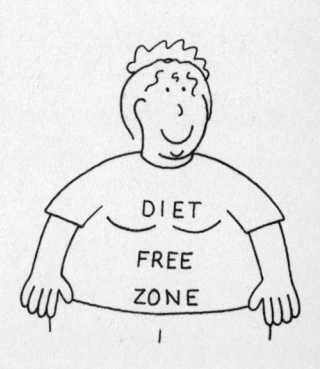

YOU KNOW YOUR DIET ISN'T WORKING WHEN . . .

You control your severe chocolate urges quite successfully...by eating a round of bacon sarnies instead.

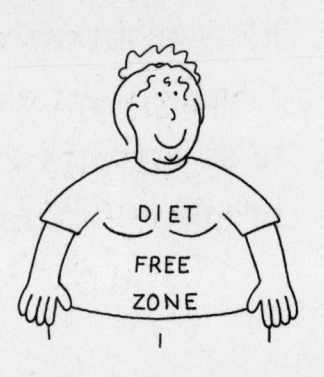

YOU KNOW YOUR DIET ISN'T WORKING WHEN . . .

Life won't be worth living when you discover that Willy Wonka's Chocolate Factory is fictitious.

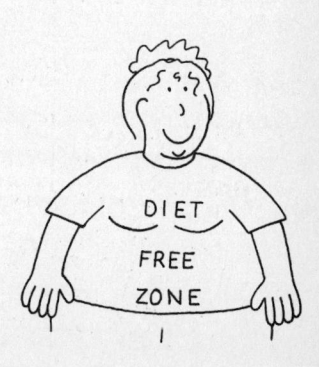

YOU KNOW YOUR DIET ISN'T WORKING WHEN . . .

Your gravity causes the Space Shuttle to fly off course.

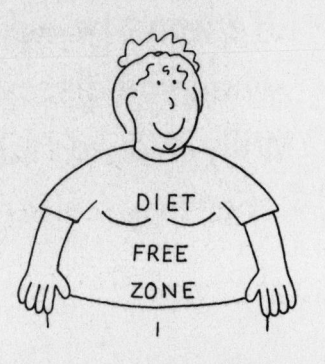

YOU KNOW YOUR DIET ISN'T WORKING WHEN . . .

You're really pleased to hear that the fuller figure is back in fashion. You'll only have to lose about 5 stone to achieve that.

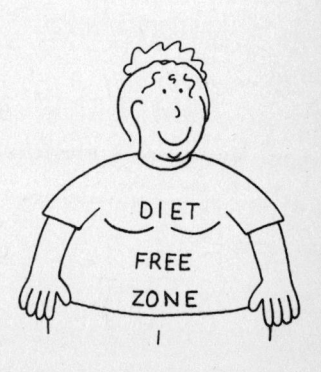

YOU KNOW YOUR DIET ISN'T WORKING WHEN . . .

If you go without food for long, you get cold turkey – in a club sandwich with mayonnaise, cheese and extra dripping.

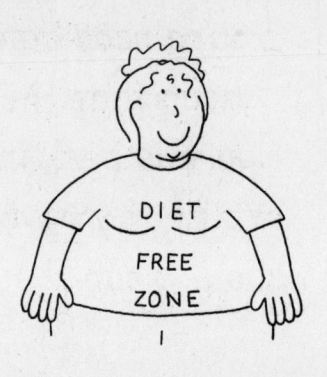

YOU KNOW YOUR DIET ISN'T WORKING WHEN . . .

In order to lose weight you donate you liver, kidneys and an arm rather than cut back on your food.

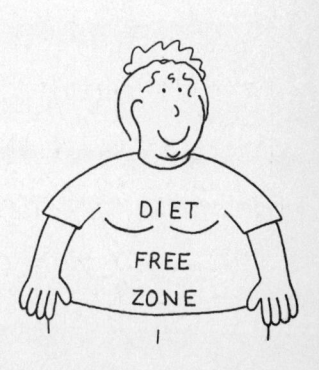

YOU KNOW YOUR DIET ISN'T WORKING WHEN . . .

You can only achieve a normal weight reading by standing on two sets of adjacent scales.

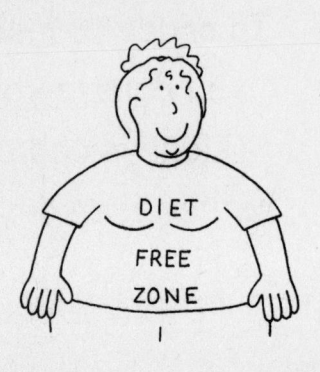

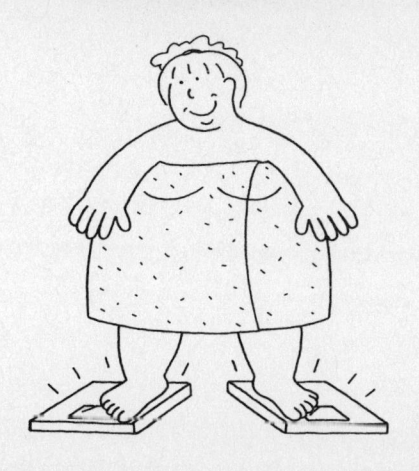

YOU KNOW YOUR DIET ISN'T WORKING WHEN . . .

Kind friends pretend to believe that you have an unfortunate thyroid problem.

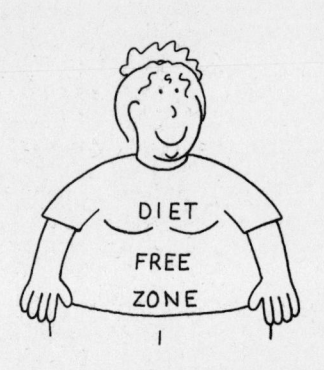

YOU KNOW YOUR DIET ISN'T WORKING WHEN . . .

You wash medicinal pills down with custard.

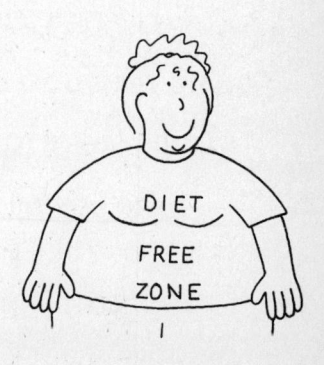

YOU KNOW YOUR DIET ISN'T WORKING WHEN . . .

You've had one of your stomachs stapled.

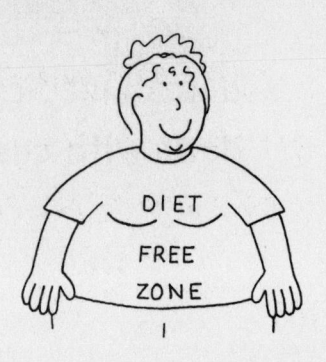

YOU KNOW YOUR DIET ISN'T WORKING WHEN . . .

Local restaurants have to restock between courses if you're dining there.

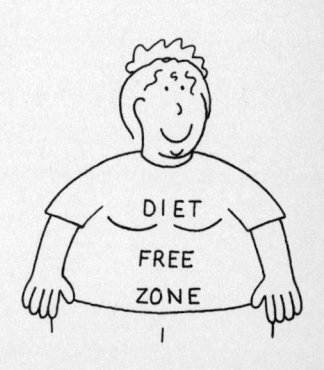

YOU KNOW YOUR DIET ISN'T WORKING WHEN . . .

You're an impatient cook...raw ingredients taste just as good if you eat enough of them.

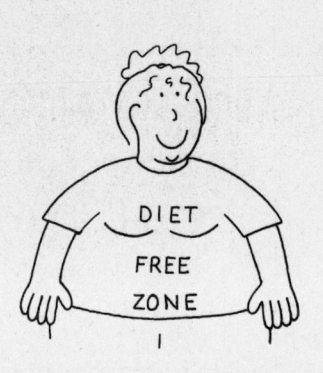

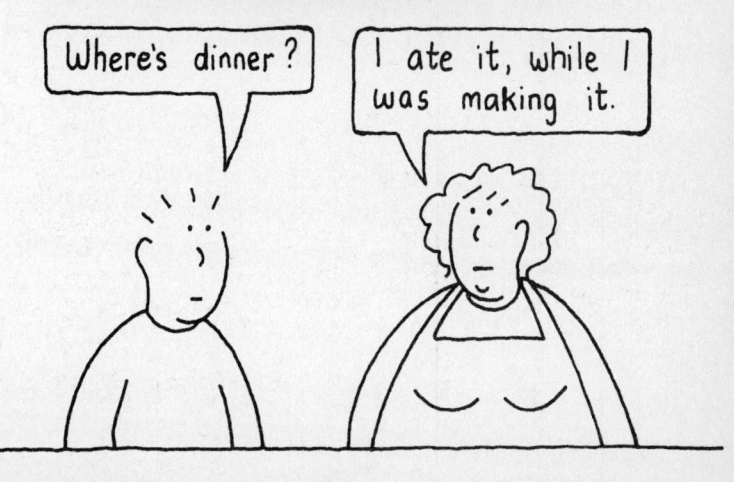

YOU KNOW YOUR DIET ISN'T WORKING WHEN . . .

You floss your teeth with bacon rind.

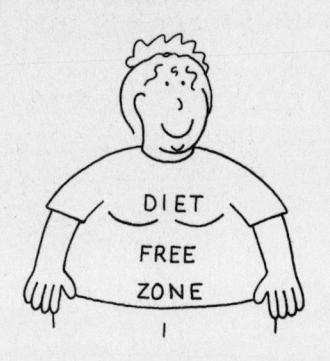

YOU KNOW YOUR DIET ISN'T WORKING WHEN . . .

You're the only person to fancy Elvis in his burger-binge days.

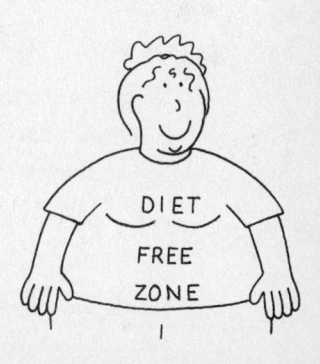

YOU KNOW YOUR DIET ISN'T WORKING WHEN . . .

You've had an operation to widen your gullet.

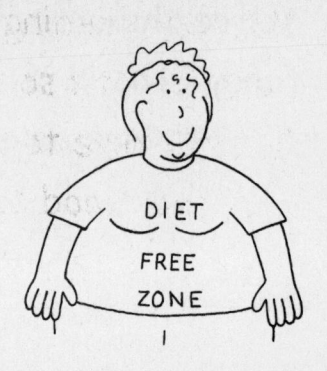

YOU KNOW YOUR DIET ISN'T WORKING WHEN . . .

You hate holding dinner parties...it's so unfair that you have to share all that food out.

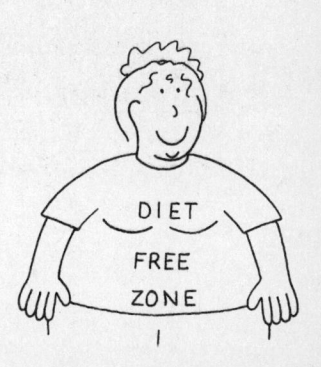

YOU KNOW YOUR DIET ISN'T WORKING WHEN . . .

Your ideal partner would be someone without the gift of sight. Or touch.

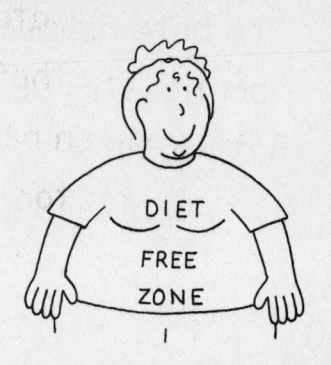

YOU KNOW YOUR DIET ISN'T WORKING WHEN . . .

You wear maternity clothes...and that applies to the men reading this too.

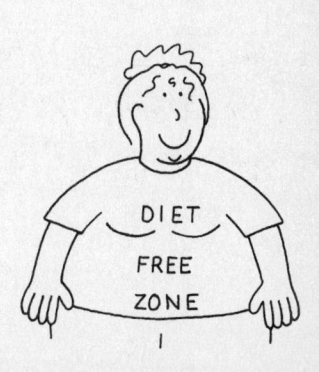

DIET FREE ZONE

YOU KNOW YOUR DIET ISN'T WORKING WHEN . . .

Having a dip at your local swimming pool causes so much water displacement that the spectators get wetter than those in the deep end.

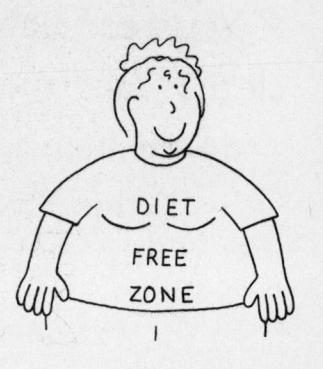

YOU KNOW YOUR DIET ISN'T WORKING WHEN . . .

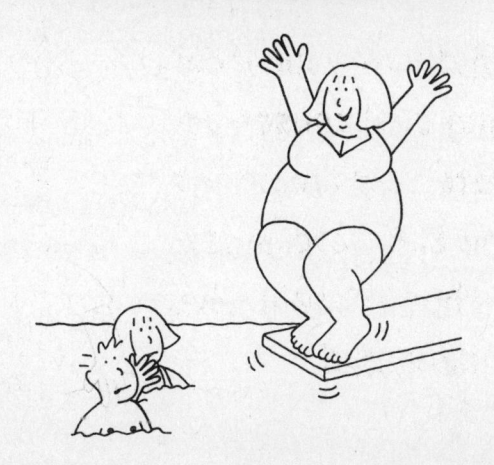

YOU KNOW YOUR DIET ISN'T WORKING WHEN . . .

You audition for the eponymous role in a film called Sea Cow. You win the part – and an Oscar.

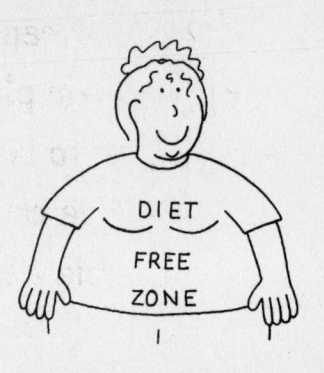

YOU KNOW YOUR DIET ISN'T WORKING WHEN . . .

A local entrepreneur applies for planning permission to build a dry ski-slope on your double chin.

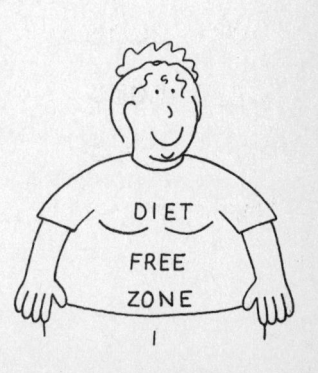

YOU KNOW YOUR DIET ISN'T WORKING WHEN . . .

You do your bit for the environment...by plugging the hole in the Ozone Layer with one of your buttocks.

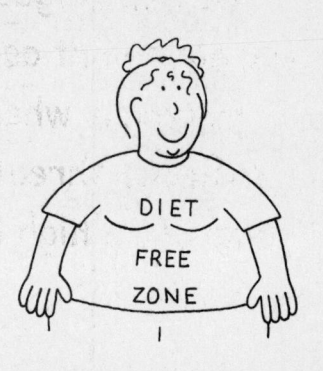

YOU KNOW YOUR DIET ISN'T WORKING WHEN . . .

The fire brigade calls you out to act as a human mattress whenever someone threatens to jump off a high building.

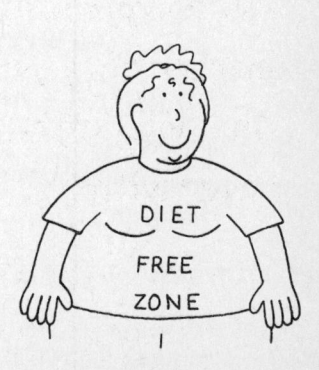

YOU KNOW YOUR DIET ISN'T WORKING WHEN . . .

As a kid you were bought a horse for Christmas, but it was more like a Shetland pony after you'd sat on it.

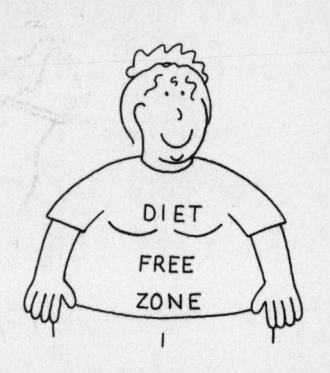

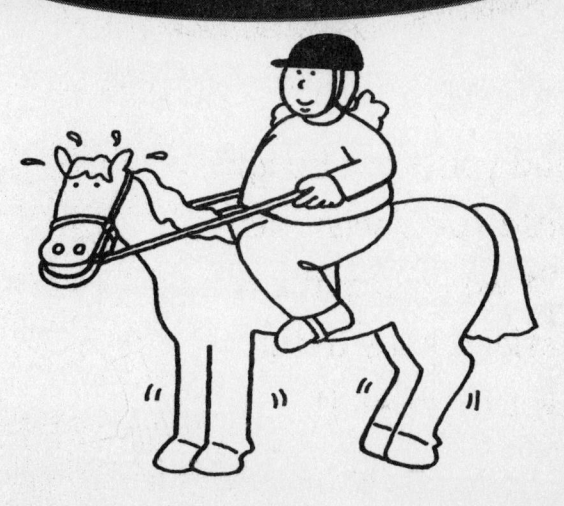

YOU KNOW YOUR DIET ISN'T WORKING WHEN . . .

Meals on Wheels refuse to deliver to you any more because you ate the wheels as well last time.

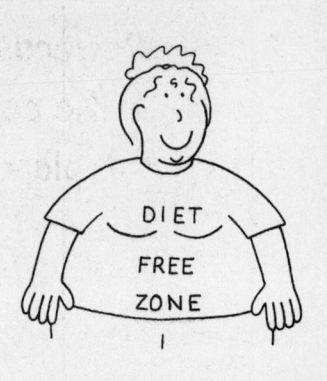

YOU KNOW YOUR DIET ISN'T WORKING WHEN . . .

Airline stewards ask you to sit in the centre of the plane.

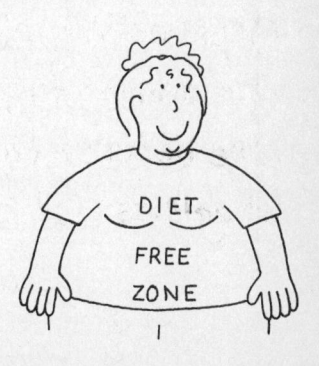

YOU KNOW YOUR DIET ISN'T WORKING WHEN . . .

You install a winch in your living room to haul your sofa out of the depression it makes in the carpet each time you sit down.

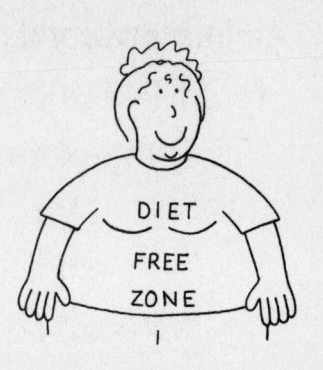

YOU KNOW YOUR DIET ISN'T WORKING WHEN . . .

You pose nude for life drawing classes, confident that no-one can see your rude bits that are conveniently concealed by the rolls of flab.

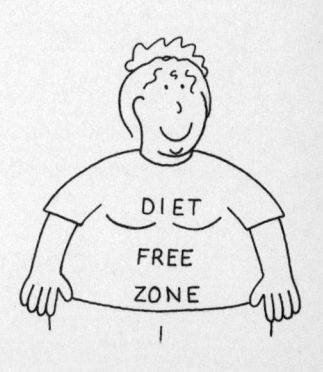

YOU KNOW YOUR DIET ISN'T WORKING WHEN . . .

You convert your home to an open-plan layout...so that you no longer have to squeeze your bulk through doorways.

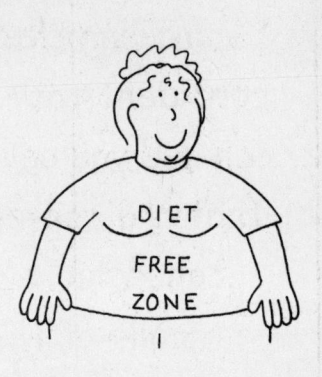

YOU KNOW YOUR DIET ISN'T WORKING WHEN . . .

You're grateful for the invention of mobile phones...you could never fit in a telephone box.

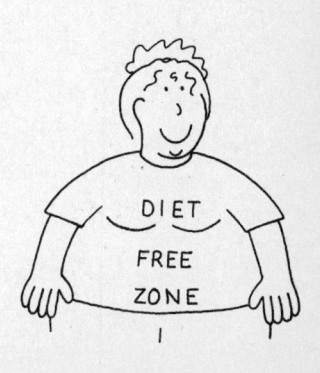

YOU KNOW YOUR DIET ISN'T WORKING WHEN . . .

Your idea of weight lifting is raising a pork pie to your mouth.

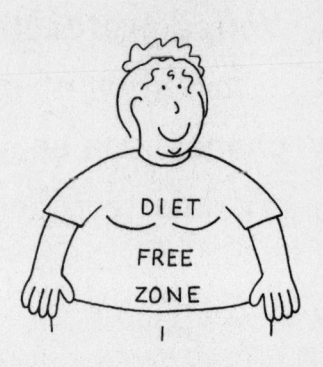

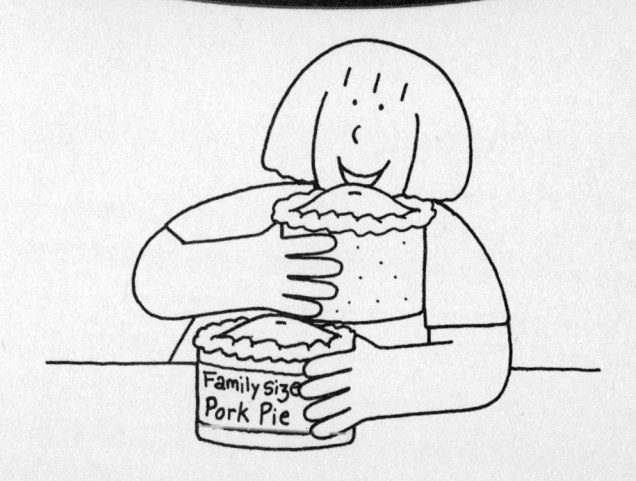

YOU KNOW YOUR DIET ISN'T WORKING WHEN . . .

You go on holiday to America where your obesity doesn't stand you out too much from the crowd.

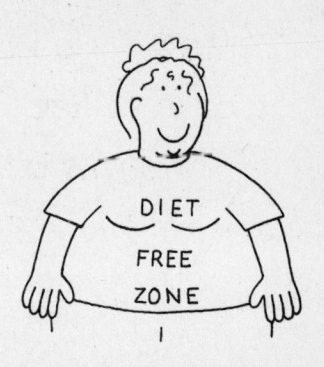

YOU KNOW YOUR DIET ISN'T WORKING WHEN . . .

You wear a leather belt...to keep your socks up.

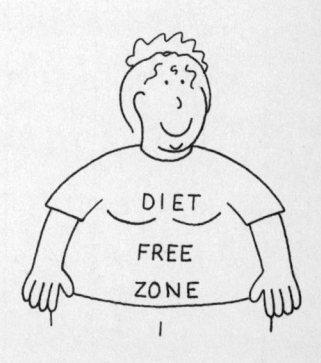

YOU KNOW YOUR DIET ISN'T WORKING WHEN . . .

You're refused entry to Venice because it's already sinking.

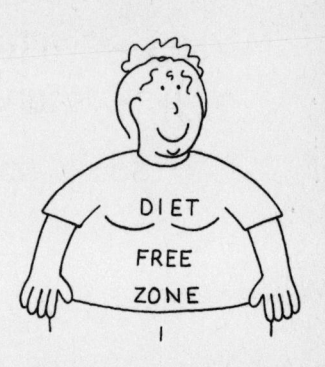

YOU KNOW YOUR DIET ISN'T WORKING WHEN . . .

The Council wants build a bypass around you.

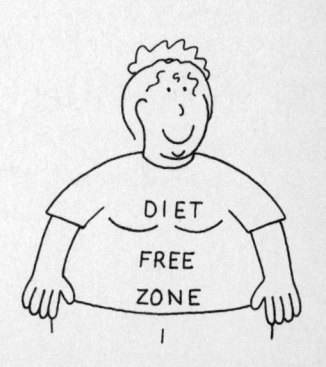

YOU KNOW YOUR DIET ISN'T WORKING WHEN . . .

You are banned from public buildings in case of fire. You might block the escape routes.

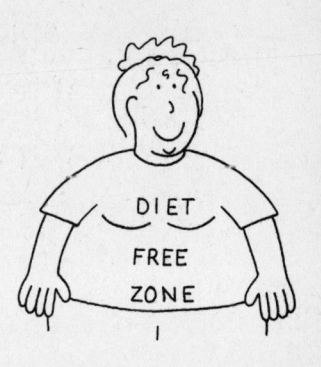

YOU KNOW YOUR DIET ISN'T WORKING WHEN . . .

You tell people you're really fit. Afterall, your jaw muscles are beautifully toned.

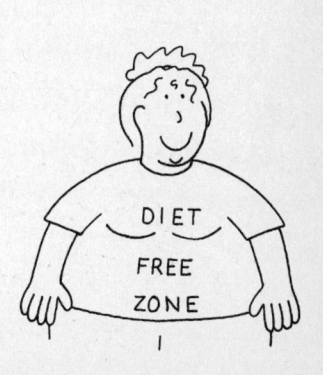

YOU KNOW YOUR DIET ISN'T WORKING WHEN . . .

Norway applies for a whaling license to extract your blubber.

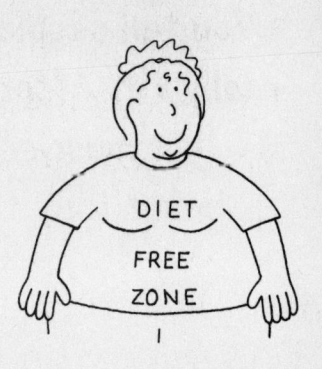

YOU KNOW YOUR DIET ISN'T WORKING WHEN . . .

You complain to the waiter if there's too much meat on your fat.

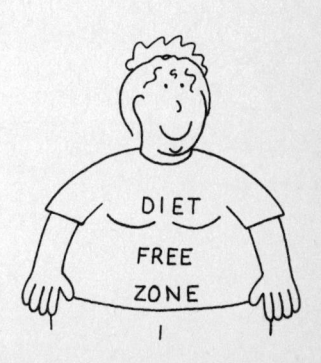

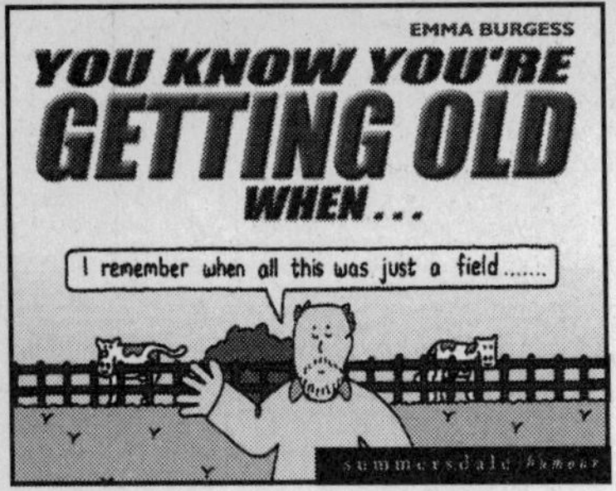
EMMA BURGESS
YOU KNOW YOU'RE GETTING OLD WHEN...
I remember when all this was just a field.......
summersdale humour

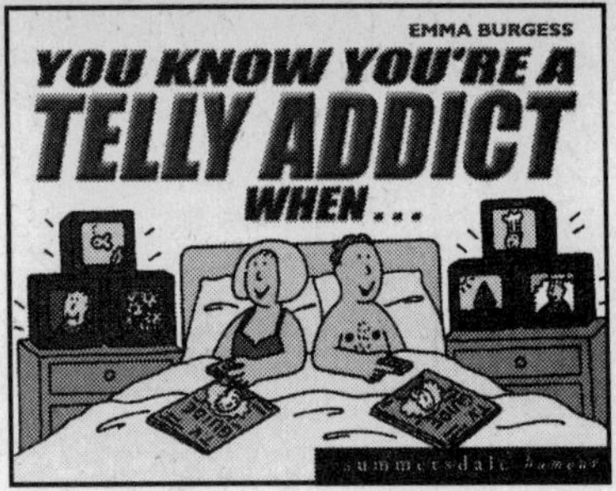
EMMA BURGESS
YOU KNOW YOU'RE A TELLY ADDICT WHEN...
summersdale humour

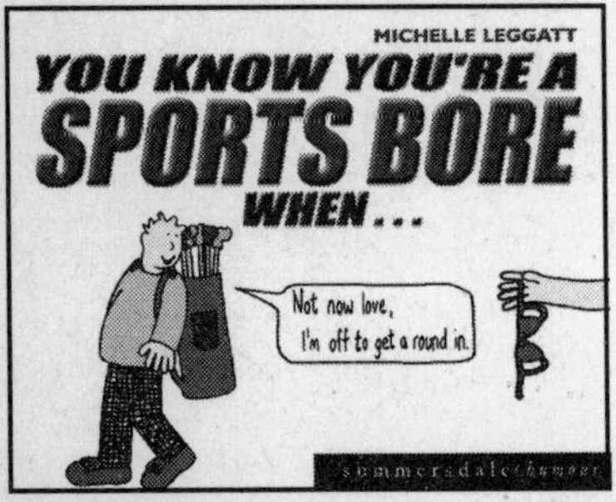
MICHELLE LEGGATT
YOU KNOW YOU'RE A SPORTS BORE WHEN...
Not now love,
I'm off to get a round in.
summersdale humour

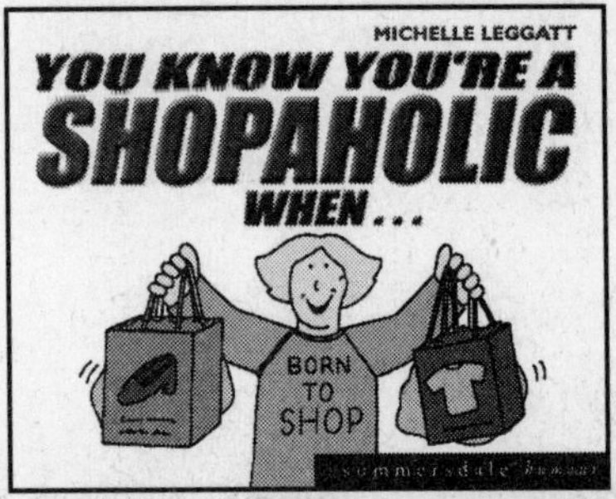
MICHELLE LEGGATT
YOU KNOW YOU'RE A SHOPAHOLIC WHEN...
BORN TO SHOP
summersdale humour

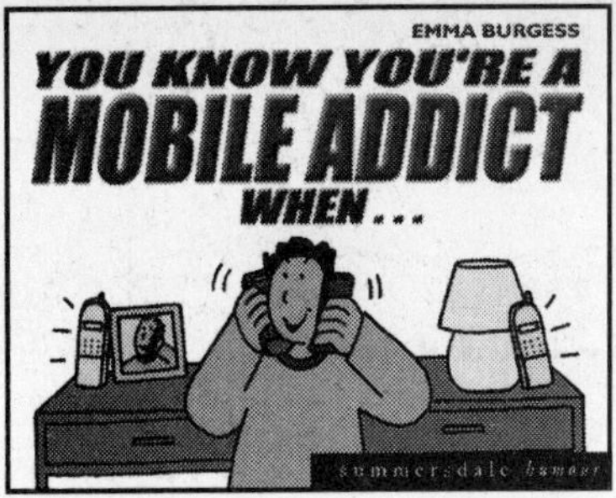
EMMA BURGESS
YOU KNOW YOU'RE A
MOBILE ADDICT
WHEN...
summersdale humour

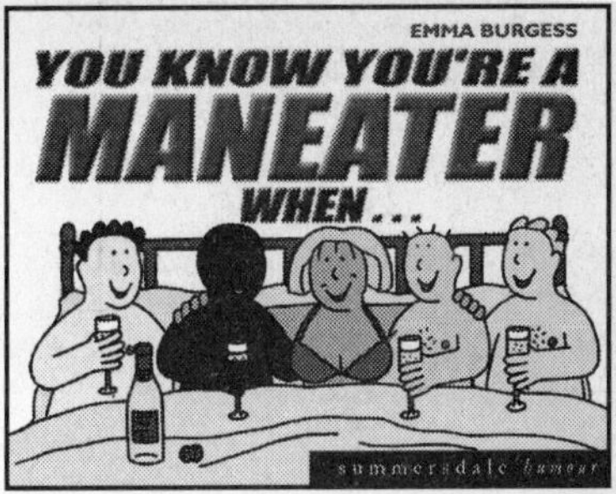
EMMA BURGESS
YOU KNOW YOU'RE A
MANEATER
WHEN...
summersdale humour

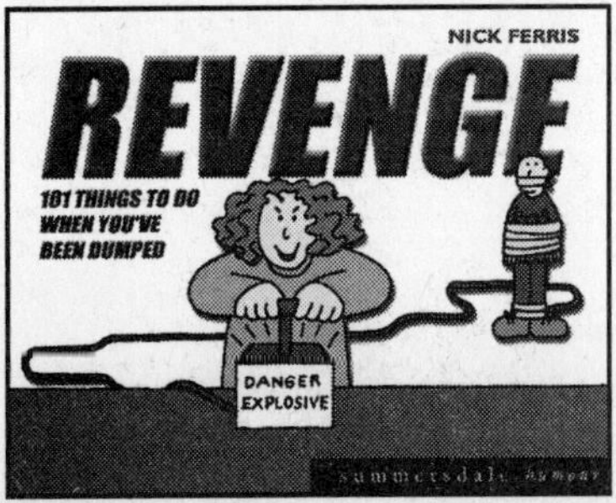
NICK FERRIS
REVENGE
101 THINGS TO DO
WHEN YOU'VE
BEEN DUMPED
DANGER
EXPLOSIVE
summersdale humour

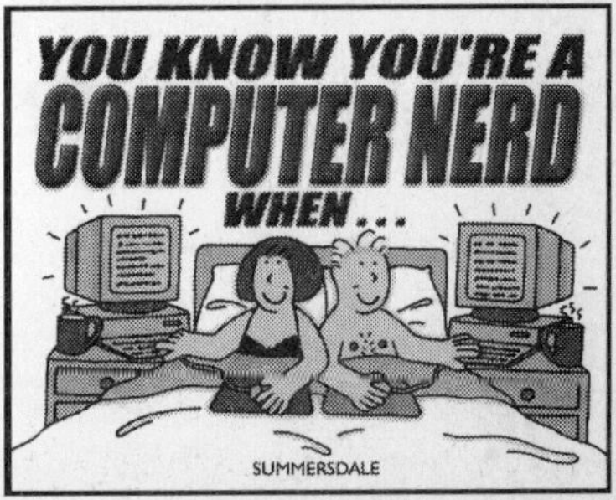
YOU KNOW YOU'RE A
COMPUTER NERD
WHEN...
SUMMERSDALE

For the latest humour books from Summersdale, check out

www.summersdale.com